A SIMPLIFIED GUIDE TO AUTONOMIC DYSFUNCTION

WHY THE BRAIN FAILS TO REPAIR ITSELF

DR. PATRICK M. NEMECHEK, D.O.
JEAN R. NEMECHEK, J.D.

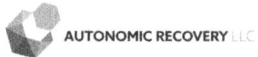

Copyright © 2017 by Autonomic Recovery, LLC.

All Rights Reserved.

Dr. Patrick M. Nemechek, D.O. and Jean R. Nemechek produced this material as work for hire.

No part of this book may be reproduced in any form or by any electronic or mechanical means, including information storage and retrieval systems, without written permission from the authors through Autonomic Recovery, LLC, except for the use of brief quotations in a book review.

Requests for permission to make copies or reproduce any part of the book should be submitted online to Request@AutonomicMed.com.

The information and the images contained within this publication are provided as an informational resource only, and are not to be used or relied on for any diagnostic or medical or treatment purposes.

This information is not intended to be patient education, and does not create any patient-physician relationship.

Please consult with a licensed healthcare practitioner to determine if any of these particular therapeutic approaches is appropriate for you or your child.

GLOSSARY

- **ALA, Alpha-Linolenic Acid** = An omega-3 fatty acid commonly supplemented in the form of nuts, flax, or chia.
- **Arachidonic Acid** = An omega-6 fatty acid that is part of the inflammation-producing process.
- **Autonomic Nervous System** = A large portion of the nervous system that regulates blood pressure, coordinates all organs (heart, intestines, bladder, etc.), controls inflammation, and regulates hormone production.
- **Bacterial Overgrowth** = Often used to refer to excessive bacterial growth within a segment of the intestinal tract. Less specific than the term SIBO, which also implies a positive methane or hydrogen breath test, or an abnormal quantification study from small intestinal aspirate.
- **CBI** = Cumulative Brain Injury. The cumulative damage that results from the residual defects remaining after improperly repaired physical, inflammatory, or metabolic damage.
- **Concussion** = A physical injury to the brain that results in persistent symptoms for several days. Also referred to as a minor traumatic brain injury or mTBI.

- **Cumulative Brain Injury** = The cumulative damage that results from the residual defects remaining after improperly repaired physical, inflammatory, or metabolic damage.
- **Cytokines, Anti-Inflammatory** = Chemicals released from white blood cells that decrease the inflammatory response.
- **Cytokines, Pro Inflammatory** = Chemicals released from white blood cells that increase the inflammatory response.
- **Developmental Delay** = The slowing of the normal rate of neurological and emotional maturation of a child. Often it is the result of excessive inflammation, nutritional deficiencies, and improper neuron pruning.
- **Developmental Arrest** = The complete stoppage of neurological and emotional maturation of a child. Often it is the result of excessive inflammation, nutritional deficiencies, and improper neuron pruning.
- **DHA** = Docosahexaenoic acid (DHA) is an omega-3 fatty acid that is a primary structural component of the human brain, cerebral cortex, skin, and retina. Dietary sources include wild fish, fish oil, and meat from animals that have fed on their natural food (e.g. grass fed beef).
- **Digestive Enzymes** = Supplements often provided to improve digestion and intestinal symptoms.
- **Dysbiosis** = Refers to a general disruption of normal microbial balance within the intestinal tract. Dysbiosis can refer to any segment of the intestinal tract (mouth, small intestine, or colon), and although it usually implies bacteria, it may also be used in regard to protozoan, fungi, or archaebacteria.
- **EPA** = Eicosapentaenoic acid (EPA) is an omega-3 fatty acid. Dietary sources include wild fish, fish oil, and meat from animals that have fed on their natural food (e.g. grass fed beef).
- **EVOO** = Extra Virgin Olive Oil. EVOO is the highest

quality of olive oil and is considered to have excellent flavor characteristics. It contains oleic acid, which is an omega-9 fatty acid.
- **Inflammation** = A normal response by the immune system to fight infection or repair damaged tissues. Excessive inflammation can lead to damaging effects in the body.
- **Intestinal Bacterial Overgrowth** = Often used when referring to the excessive presence of bacteria within the small intestine. These bacteria often originate in the colon (lower or large intestine) and abnormally migrate up to the small intestine.
- **Inulin** = A prebiotic fiber that is preferentially digested by the types of bacteria that normally inhabit the small intestine.
- **Linolenic Acid** = An omega-6 fatty acid that is part of the inflammation-producing process. Commonly found in plants and in high concentrations within a wide variety of cooking oils.
- **Microglia, M0** = These are a specialized form of white blood cell that live in the brain. They are often referred to as surveillance or pruning microglia.
- **Microglia, M1** - These are a specialized form of white blood cell that live in the brain. They promote inflammation and are part of the healthy repair process but can cause damage if they become primed.
- **Microglia, M2** - These are a specialized form of white blood cell that live in the brain. They shut off inflammation and are part of the healthy repair process.
- **Microglia, Primed** = These are microglia that permanently morph into M1-microglia and prevent the brain from fully repairing brain traumas. They also are a major source of inflammatory cytokines within the brain.
- **mTBI** = Minor (lower case letter M) traumatic brain injury.

This is a brain injury that is relatively mild, and is commonly referred to as concussion.
- **MTBI** = Major (upper case letter M) traumatic brain injury. A brain injury that has caused significant cellular damage and is often associated with intracranial bleeding.
- **Neuron** = A cell within the brain that carries or stores neurological information.
- **Neuroplasticity** = The process through which the brain develops new neuronal pathways to perform certain tasks.
- **Oleic Acid** = An omega-9 fatty acid that is very plentiful in olive oil. Oleic acid blocks the brain damage that can result from excessive omega-6 fatty acids and palmitic acid.
- **Omega-3 Fatty Acid** = These nutrients are unsaturated fatty acids and are important for normal metabolism. They are classified as an essential nutrient because humans are unable to synthesize omega-3 fatty acids, and require them in their diet in order to remain healthy.
- **Omega-6 Fatty Acid** = These nutrients are a family of pro-inflammatory and anti-inflammatory polyunsaturated fatty acids. They are commonly found in plants and are classified as essential nutrients.
- **Omega-9 Fatty Acid** = These are unsaturated fatty acids and are not essential nutrients. Oleic acid, found within olive oil, is an example of an omega-9 fatty acid.
- **Palmitic Acid** = This nutrient is the most common saturated fatty acid found in animals, plants, and microorganisms; excessive amounts in human diet results in an increase of inflammation within the brain.
- **Phenotype** = A phenotype is the visible characteristic of how an animal, cell, or plant looks or behaves. (Genotype is the potential characteristic coded in the organism's DNA).
- **Prebiotic** = A form of fiber that induces the growth or activity of beneficial microorganisms (e.g. bacteria and

fungi). The most common example is in the gastrointestinal tract where the digestion of prebiotic fibers can alter the composition of organisms in the gut microbiome.
- **Probiotic** = Bacterial organisms that are ingested or added to foods, and are potentially beneficial to health.
- **Propionic Acid** = A small chain fatty acid produced by bacteria within the intestinal tract.
- **RifaGut**™ = Another market brand name for rifaximin.
- **Rifaximin** = The generic term for the non-absorbable antibiotic sold under the brand names Xifaxan™, Rifagut™, Rifaximina™ and SIBOFix™.
- **SIBO** = Small Intestine Bacterial Overgrowth. A specific form of bacterial overgrowth, which is designated by a positive methane or hydrogen breath test, or an abnormal quantification study from small intestinal aspirate.
- **SIBOFix**™ = Another market brand name for rifaximin.
- **Synapse** = A portion of a neuron (or nerve cell) that permits the neuron to pass an electrical or chemical signal to another neuron.
- **The Nemechek Protocol**™ = a medical treatment program invented by Dr. Patrick M. Nemechek, D.O. relating to methods for preventing, reducing, or reversing acute and/or chronic autonomic damage by the suppression of pro-inflammatory cytokines, which is useful in treating a variety of diseases or conditions. (Patent Pending)
- **Toxic Encephalopathy** = The medical state of a child whose brain has essentially been drugged with excessive propionic acid.
- **Traumatic Brain Injury, TBI** = The term for a physical injury to the head and which results in symptoms lasting for more than 24 hours. See mTBI and MTBI.
- **Vagus Nerve** = The 10th cranial nerve of the human body

that carries the signals in the parasympathetic branch of the autonomic nervous system.
- **Vagus Nerve Stimulation, VNS** = This is a medical treatment that involves delivering electrical impulses to the Vagus nerve in the autonomic nervous system. Therapeutically VNS reduces inflammation throughout the brain and body and is capable of inducing neuroplasticity.
- **White Blood Cells (WBC)** = Cells of the immune system are often referred to as white blood cells or WBCs.
- **Xifaxan^{TM}** = This is the brand name of a time-released formulation of rifaximin sold within the United States.

ABOUT THE AUTHORS

I can explain the underlying cause of most diseases in just 13 words: "The failure of our brains sets into motion the failure of our bodies".

— Dr. Patrick M. Nemechek, D.O.

About the Authors

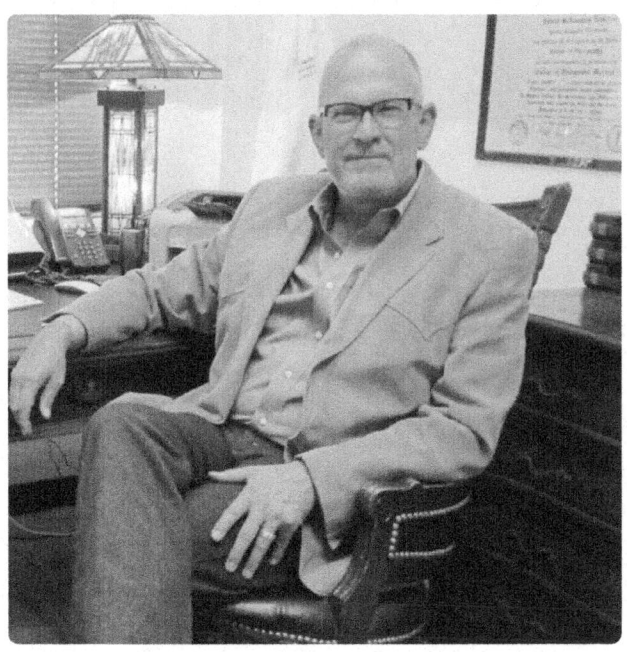

Dr. Patrick M. Nemechek, D.O. was born in Tucson, Arizona. He graduated with a B.S. in Microbiology from San Diego University (1982), and obtained his Doctorate in Osteopathic Medicine from the University of Health Sciences, Kansas City, Missouri (1987).

Dr. Nemechek completed his training in internal medicine at UCLA School of Medicine (1990), where he had the distinguished honor of being named Chief Resident and later Clinical Instructor for the Department of Medicine at UCLA.

Dr. Nemechek's mentor at UCLA was Albert Einstein's nephew, who encouraged him to go into the particularly complex field of HIV Medicine, which was the medical mystery of that time. Here Dr. Nemechek would have the challenging freedom to save people's lives.

While at UCLA, Dr. Nemechek was recognized with the awarding of the Robert S. Mosser Award for Excellence in Internal Medicine, for his outstanding academic performance and instrumental role in starting UCLA's first HIV clinic at Kern Medical Center, Bakersfield, California.

In 1994, Dr. Nemechek moved to Kansas City, Missouri, where he opened an HIV treatment and research facility named Nemechek Health Renewal.

It was at this point that Dr. Nemechek started work in earnest, as a classically trained internal medicine "scientist-physician", entering the field of HIV at a time when there were no diagnostic tests, no treatments, and no answers.

Those early decades transformed Dr. Nemechek into an innovator who followed the latest research, looked at problems at a cellular and metabolic level, and became one of the first doctors to figure out ways to treat wasting syndrome, as well as other complex HIV-related problems.

Dr. Nemechek's innovative approach to the complexities of HIV disease garnered him many honors, such as being chosen as a "Site of Clinical Excellence" by Bristol Myers Squibb Company & KPMG Peat Marwick, being named as one of the top HIV physicians in the U.S. by POZ magazine and receiving several nominations for the Small Business of the Year Awards by the Greater Kansas City Chamber of Commerce.

During his 20 years in the Midwest, Dr. Nemechek authored or collaborated on 72 scientific abstracts, publications, or posters and he participated in 41 different clinical studies. In 1999 he became a founding investigator for the HIV Research Network, a consortium of 18 different universities and HIV treatment facilities, funded by the U.S. Department of Health and Human Services.

He has served on numerous editorial, professional, and advisory boards as well as founding two non-profit HIV health advocacy organizations, the Bakersfield Aids Foundation and Fight Back KC.

By 2004, many of Dr. Nemechek's HIV patients were stable, and leading normal lives, but strangely they were starting to die of sudden cardiac events due to Cardiac Autonomic Neuropathy (CAN). Dr. Nemechek set out to learn more about this lethal phenomenon, and in 2006 purchased a new technology, called spectral analysis, which allowed him to tune into the communication signals between the heart and the brain, quantifying the balance and tone of these two branches of the autonomic nervous system.

Dr. Nemechek received additional training in autonomic testing and analysis at the Universidade De Lisboa, in Lisbon, Portugal, one of the top autonomic research facilities in the world.

Dr. Nemechek has now performed and analyzed thousands of autonomic patterns of damage. The more Dr. Nemechek learned about the field of Autonomic Medicine, the more he realized that it is the failure of the brain that sets into motion the failure of the body.

With his extensive research experience and expertise in metabolism, immunology, and the autonomic nervous system, Dr. Nemechek returned to his home state of Arizona in 2010, with his wife Jean, and opened Nemechek Consultative Medicine, an Internal Medicine and Autonomic Medicine practice.

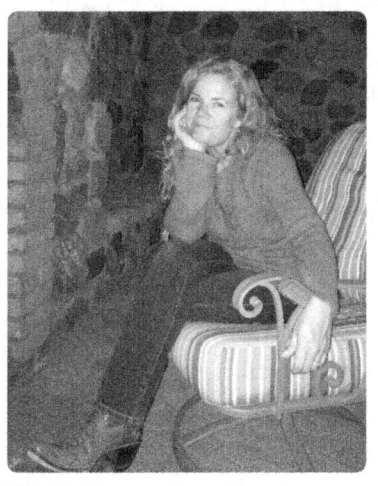

Jean Nemechek is uniquely qualified to run the business, and co-author with, Dr. Nemechek as she graduated with a B.A. in Communications and a B.S. in Journalism from the University of Kansas (1988, 1989) and a Juris Doctorate from Washburn School of Law (1993).

After relocating back home to Arizona, Dr. Nemechek was once again treating children and adults of all ages for routine matters. He was shocked at how incredibly sick the general population had become in just a few decades.

The disease continuum had moved up about 40 years it seemed, and diseases that had once struck only the elderly were routinely occurring in middle age or early adulthood.

Dr. Nemechek could recall when he was a medical student and his instructor had called him into an exam room to see a person in their 50's who had diabetes. It was unheard of in those days to have someone "so young" with type II diabetes. Tragically that disease is now quite commonplace in middle age, as we have become collectively sick and old at an accelerated pace.

Dr. Nemechek realized that many of his routine patients were suffering from the early stages of disease and autonomic dysfunction (heartburn, headaches, fatigue), small intestine bacterial overgrowths – SIBO (intestinal distress, food intolerances), and their children were also increasingly experiencing the symptoms arising from autonomic dysfunction and SIBO (anxiety, ADD, autism, and digestive and intestinal issues).

This is where Dr. Nemechek began, once again, to make history. He knew he had to change the practice of modern medicine back to the goals of healing the patient and reversing disease.

Dr. Nemechek began to approach his regular patients with same the investigative research angle that he had done with HIV, he pushed beyond the disease labels to understand and resolve the underlying problems.

Dr. Nemechek started using all available scientific and medical tools to induce the nervous system and organs to repair themselves by normalizing inflammation control mechanisms, inducing natural stem cell production, and reactivating innate restorative mechanisms.

Starting in 2010, Dr. Nemechek embarked on an extraordinary path that involved altering and improving intestinal bacteria and reducing pro-inflammatory cytokines within the central nervous system, and he witnessed unprecedented recovery in all five stages of autonomic dysfunction without long-term medication. This was unheard of in our time.

As the years passed Dr. Nemechek also began working with various current and former professional athletes whose brain symptoms he resolved (Autonomic Advantage™ Brain Injury Recovery Program), offered expert opinions on Autonomic Medicine in the United States Court of Federal Claims, and he began incorporating bioelectric medicine, specifically electro-modulation of the Vagus nerve, with his patients.

Dr. Nemechek found the key to treatment and reversal of many of the common diseases affecting people today is by reversing the dysfunction of the autonomic nervous system in combination with the renewal of stem cell production and neurogenesis, through the reduction of metabolic inflammation.

Because of his efforts and career experiences, Dr. Nemechek invented an effective program to prevent, reduce, or reverse autonomic nervous system damage through a combination of natural neurochemical supplements, short-term prescription medications, dietary restrictions, and neuromodulation of the Vagus nerve.

Dr. Nemechek's treatment approach is extremely effective in the recovery of autonomic functions from a variety of neuroinflammatory conditions including traumatic brain injury, concussion, chronic traumatic encephalopathy (CTE), post-concussion syndrome (PCS), Alzheimer's disease, Parkinson's disease, essential tremors, post-traumatic stress disorder (PTSD), chronic depression, treatment resistant epilepsy, autism, developmental delays, Asperger's syndrome, and sensory and motor disorders.

In 2016, Dr. Nemechek filed a patent application to protect his groundbreaking formula that is now known as "The Nemechek Protocol™" or The Nemechek Protocol™ for Autonomic Recovery (Patent Pending).

In response to his unique expertise in clinical autonomics and the development of The Nemechek Protocol™ for Autonomic Recovery (Patent Pending), the practice was renamed Nemechek Autonomic Medicine in 2017.

This book is an introduction to the main problems and symptoms associated with autonomic dysfunction, and the contributing factor of intestinal bacterial overgrowth to brain injury and recovery.

By applying certain parts of The Nemechek Protocol™ to treat such autonomic dysfunction and intestinal bacterial overgrowth in children, Dr. Nemechek made a breakthrough discovery in his work with autistic and developmental delay patients. His approach with these patients is now also commonly referred to as "The Nemechek Protocol™ for Autism", and it has spread throughout the world.

INTRODUCTION
ATTEMPTING THE IMPOSSIBLE – THE HISTORY OF THE NEMECHEK PROTOCOL

The research that eventually lead to The Nemechek Protocol™ started over a decade ago in an attempt to do what was considered impossible, reverse the symptoms and underlying chronic autonomic dysfunction that commonly persist after common concussion or traumatic brain injuries.

Even today, the general consensus in field of neuroscience is that the reversal of post-traumatic autonomic dysfunction greater that a few months duration is impossible.

Conferences will have presentation after presentation discussing the anatomical and symptomatic features of a variety of autonomic dysfunctions without a single presentation discussing techniques or efforts at recovery.

Patients are given impressive sounding diagnoses such as neurogenic orthostatic hypotension or postural orthostatic tachycardia syndrome (POTS), and whose symptoms are then managed with hydrates, salt, support hoses and a variety of stimulants. No therapies are directed at reversing the damage at the heart of the patient's symptoms.

For example, if an individual has persistent symptoms for more than a few months after a common sports-related concussion, they are told further recovery is impossible and are given the diagnosis of post-concussion syndrome.

But concussions are extremely common not only in sports but arise from accidents that occur in every aspect of daily life. Furthermore, most people seem to fully recover from these injuries without any residual symptoms.

Why Does One Person Recover but Not The Other?

The real problem is that 2 individuals may sustain identical injuries to their head, and experience the same set of symptoms after the injury, yet one will fully recover and the other will not.

This being the case, then the answer to the persistent symptoms lies in the inability of one person to recover from an injury and not from the injury itself. In other words, one person can repair the damage, whereas the other person cannot.

Fixing the repair process is the key to helping people repair commonplace damage to their brains.

Over the course of many years, Dr. Nemechek tested a wide variety of dietary supplements, eating patterns, exercise regimens and medications in an attempt to reverse chronic underlying autonomic damage and all failed.

Over and over again, a new combination of treatment elements was prescribed to volunteers, and objective measurements over a series of months were taken.

For several years, nothing resulted in any meaningful improvement in the patients' underlying autonomic dysfunction.

The turning point was the rising general consensus within the neuroscience community that human adults actually produced stem cells and neuroprogenitor cells within the central nervous system, and that inflammation seemed to prevent stem cells from functioning correctly.

Stem cells and neuroprogenitor cells are both unique in that they are capable of replacing or rebuilding damaged neurons within the central nervous system.

Prior to this shift in our understanding, the prevailing dogma held that all stem cell production in humans abruptly ceased at the time of birth. Many readers may recall the political and ethical debates that occurred over the use of fetal tissue for stem cell research.

Around the same time, studies were demonstrating that intravenous infusions of stems failed to provide any substantial benefit in stroke victims, because of high levels of pro-inflammatory chemicals within the subjects' blood stream.

More precisely known as pro-inflammatory cytokines, these chemicals prevented the infused stem cells from functioning within the body.

In parallel to these important findings were 2 other facts. First, since the early 1990's, it seemed the U.S. was in the midst of an epidemic of failed concussion recovery.

Secondly, scientific evidence was suggesting that the entire U.S. population was developing an abnormal inflammatory condition later referred to as 'inflamm-aging'.

The same pro-inflammatory cytokines that prevented stems from functioning were now being detected within the blood stream of seemingly healthy individuals and these levels seemed to be increasing as we aged.

Dr. Nemechek began theorizing that the increased 'inflamm-aging' of the population could possibly be interfering with their natural stem cell production and function, and might be responsible for the inability of many individuals to recovery from common concussion.

Furthermore, many of the symptoms individuals experience from their concussion are symptoms that result directly from autonomic damage.

Normalization of Inflammatory Cytokines is the Key

From this point forward, Dr. Nemechek's efforts to restore autonomic function then shifted towards trying to restore the normal neurological repair mechanisms, by reducing inflammation and increasing natural stem cell function.

The original anti-inflammatory protocol involved the use of a common omega-3 fatty acid blend of fish oil (EPA>>DHA) along with curcumin and inulin fiber, and for the first time in many years, evidence of reversal of autonomic dysfunction, as measured by spectral analysis, was seen, especially within younger patients.

Although the improvement was minor, it was significant enough to warrant further testing of other combinations.

With this success, the push was on to find to other more effective approaches to further reduce pro-inflammatory cytokine levels in order to increase the speed and degree of autonomic recovery in patients of all ages. Group after group of Dr. Nemechek's patients trialed a variety of different anti-inflammatory regimens.

After a few years of more research, Dr. Nemechek discovered that potent neurological recovery could be achieved with a very particular combination of treatment elements that are the backbone of The Nemechek ProtocolTM.

Brain injury and autonomic recovery requires the combined potency of a few critical elements, the restoration of the intestinal bacterial balance, along with an improvement in natural omega-3 and omega-6 fatty acids, that make up a large portion of every cell membrane in the body, especially the nervous system. Equally important, was that this potent regimen was inexpensive and could be achieved with a short course of antibiotics, as well as daily doses of common nutritional supplements

However, the most important discovery was the use of bioelectrical stimulation of the vagus nerve commonly referred to as vagus nerve stimulation or VNS.

VNS can be done by surgically implanted devices within the chest of an individual, or non-invasively by applying an imperceptible electrical current over a certain area of the ear. The current passes through the skin and activates the auricular branch of the vagus nerve in a process now referred to as transcutaneous auricular vagus nerve stimulation or taVNS (thank goodness for abbreviations).

taVNS is rapidly becoming a critically important tool in the reversal of a wide variety of neurological conditions and is being shown to have an effect equivalent to the more costly and invasive surgical VNS.

Interestingly, VNS has several aspects that support the reversal of chronic autonomic dysfunction as well as other forms of chronic brain damage.

Through a mechanism referred to as the cholinergic anti-inflammatory pathway (CAP), taVNS, in combination with the other components of The Nemechek ProtocolTM, reduces inflammation not only within the central nervous system, but also throughout the entire body.

As part of The Nemechek ProtocolTM, taVNS greatly increases the speed and extent of symptomatic recovery from autonomic dysfunction, even if the symptoms have been present for decades.

Coincidentally, taVNS also improves symptomatic relief from a variety inflammatory arthritic conditions and autoimmune disorders and is proving very effective in reversing a variety of psychiatric-inflammatory disorders including chronic depression, OCD, generalized anxiety and PTSD (post-traumatic stress disorder).

Lastly, the bioelectric stimulation of the vagus nerve is capable of inducing a recovery phenomenon known as neuroplasticity.

Neuroplasticity is the process through which neurons of the brain are routed or re-wired in order to restore lost functions to a limb, or autonomic capacity, or in the case of a young child, to develop a new skill such as speech, a motor function or sensory perception.

Animal and human studies are showing improvements in stroke recovery when VNS is combined with rehabilitation exercises.

Even more exciting, is that further recovery from past strokes is possible, even when these recovery efforts take place more than a year past the original date of the stroke.

After several refusals by different conferences, Dr. Nemechek's groundbreaking research was finally presented at the 13th International Neuromodulation Conference in Edinburgh, Scotland in June, 2107, and submission of his findings for publication in a peer-reviewed journal is anticipated in 2018.

1
THE IMPORTANCE OF THE AUTONOMIC NERVOUS SYSTEM

MODERN DISEASES ARE FROM AUTONOMIC NERVOUS SYSTEM DYSFUNCTION

Understanding whether you have autonomic nervous system dysfunction is often the key to many of your medical mysteries.

The reversal of a wide range of symptoms, illnesses, and chronic diseases by repairing your cellular, brain, and nervous system damage is a new and whole-body approach to medicine. To fix the body, we must fix the brain.

Modern illnesses often begin with subtle changes in how our brain is able to coordinate and regulate our body.

When our autonomic nervous system begins to malfunction we get headaches, heartburn, feel lightheaded or dizzy, feel anxious, have abnormal heart rhythms, or experience intestinal trouble. We may need to go to the bathroom more often, experience chronic pain or chronic fatigue, or we just feel "off".

Autonomic dysfunction makes it more difficult to wake up in the morning, or it may be more difficult for us to go to sleep, or to stay asleep, at night. We may fidget, cannot focus, and feel anxious.

The autonomics also control many small functions like our pupils' ability to respond to bright sunlight without needing sunglasses, being able to see while driving at night, sweating, and temperature regulation.

When the autonomics malfunction it can makes us feel too hungry, and thus contributes to obesity due to the false need to snack during the day for what we believe are "low blood sugar" symptoms.

Autonomic dysfunction can also produce abnormal hunger a few hours after having a full meal and the stress hormones contribute to stubborn belly fat.

Early autonomic dysfunction in adults includes high blood pressure, sleep apnea or insomnia, and cerebral blood flow issues that leave them with ADD, dizziness, brain fog, memory problems, and anxiety.

Today's young adults and children are also experiencing a great deal of autonomic dysfunction. They are increasingly unable to heal from concussions, they have gastrointestinal and digestion trouble, and they are developing ADD/ADHD, autism, and anxiety.

Learning about the signs and stages of autonomic dysfunction may help you finally get to the underlying cause of your medical issues and provide a framework for you to regain your health.

Improving and reversing autonomic dysfunction is important for people of all ages because, when the autonomics malfunction for long enough, the resulting metabolic inflammation will ultimately help to turn on someone's genetic system for disease creation.

WHAT IS THE AUTONOMIC NERVOUS SYSTEM?

The autonomic nervous system is the main communications network between the brain and the heart, the organs, the digestive tract, the lungs, and as well as the immune system and hormonal regulation.

When your autonomics work correctly they are "automatic" and you do not even know they exist. The autonomics encompass almost everything that goes wrong when your body is not working "automatically", and perfectly, as it should.

The nerves within the autonomics are the brain's master control mechanism for the body. The field of autonomics is not a new area of medicine but until recently autonomics were only explored in research studies and labs, more fascinating to watch and study than for practical use in fighting common or complex illnesses.

The autonomic branches were also too complex to be tested in regular outpatient settings and doctors did not know how to repair them once they had malfunctioned.

Advances in medical technology are making autonomic testing available in regular medical offices like mine, and I have discovered treatment methods for autonomic improvement, or repair, without the use of long-term medications that only stabilize or mask a symptom. These things will help to open up the field of autonomics and move it into modern primary care.

The autonomics control every organ in the body such as the heart, bladder, stomach, intestines, and kidneys. It is how the brain regulates your blood pressure, blood sugar levels, sleep cycles, immune system, and your hormones.

The autonomics also control many smaller functions such as when your pupils dilate, when you have hiccups, and the adrenaline that produces nightmares. Basic bodily functions that no one really thinks about until the moment they start to malfunction.

The autonomics also coordinate our emotionality and how intensely we react to stressors. The same forces that damage the autonomics may also damage other areas of the brain and produce the symptoms of anxiety, depression, and PTSD.

HOW DOES THE AUTONOMIC NERVOUS SYSTEM WORK?

The autonomic nervous system communicates and coordinates the metabolic state of the cells in the human body through two main branches. One is the sympathetic nervous system (sympathetic) and the other is the parasympathetic nervous system (parasympathetic).

In simple terms, the sympathetic branch is responsible for energy expenditure ("fight or flight") and the parasympathetic branch is responsible for energy conservation and restoration ("rest and digest").

The sympathetic branch controls the body's response to stress, pain, and cold. The parasympathetic branch controls the body's resting state after a meal, at night, the digestive tract, nutrient storage, immune responses, and healing.

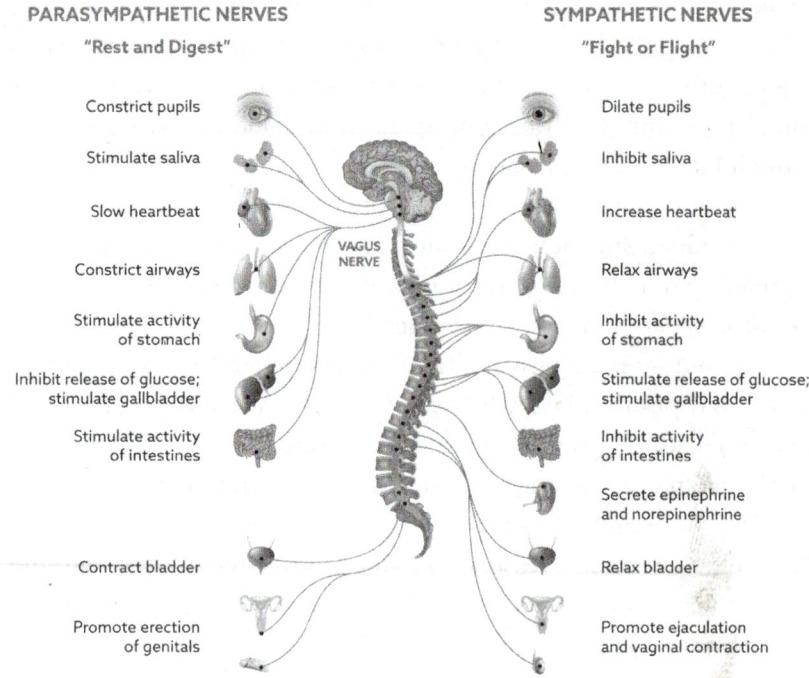

If the sympathetic commands are disrupted people may feel tired, crave salt or sugar, experience excessive hunger, or get anxious. People may get heart palpitations, tingling or numbness in their arms (hands or face), disrupted night vision, varicose veins, erectile dysfunction, stiff necks and shoulders, or severe ("migraine") headaches.

Sympathetic dysfunction may also create adrenaline rushes that fuel insomnia, nightmares, aggression, or anger.

If the parasympathetic commands are disrupted they may affect the intestinal tract (heartburn or constipation), the immune system (autoimmune disorders), or produce chronic pain syndromes (fibromyalgia).

These people may get sleep apnea, "restless legs", morning nausea, night sweats or hot flushes, intolerance to light because of dilated pupils, or feel power surge sensations when they should be at rest. Parasympathetic dysfunction may leave them exhausted in the morning despite a full night of sleep.

Both the sympathetic and parasympathetic branches feed into the heart and modulate the heart's natural rhythms and ability of the heart muscle to contract.

Damage or disruption to the function of either of these branches causes a wide variety of symptoms to occur, and many people experience both sympathetic and parasympathetic branch symptoms.

These two opposite autonomic branches should work together simultaneously and in balance, which is called sympathovagal balance. When these two autonomic branches are in balance the body works automatically and a person feels no symptoms.

Without proper balance one branch may become withdrawn or the other becomes elevated. When the branches are no longer working automatically, a person may feel symptoms that range from mild (feeling dizzy or a getting a head rush when standing up from a chair) to completely debilitating (falling or passing out).

Sympathovagal balance between the sympathetic and parasympathetic branches is not just important for feeling better in the short term; sympathovagal balance is necessary for a long and healthy life.

When the sympathetic and parasympathetic branches are not in sympathovagal balance, and if left untreated, the imbalance will result in a loss of heart rate variability (HRV), which is associated with increased mortality from all causes.

Improved autonomic function improves heart rate variability (HRV), which is the time interval between heartbeats.

People with elevated HRV have an increased risk of developing atrial fibrillation or heart flutter. People with low HRV have an increased risk of widespread organ and metabolic dysfunction.

Autonomic dysfunction also fuels the systemic metabolic inflammation that triggers cellular changes and ignites someone's disposition for diseases (cancer, diabetes, hypertension, etc.).

This is why my goal, as a physician, is to improve and restore autonomic functioning because it is critical to life expectancy.

2
AUTONOMIC DYSFUNCTION

WHAT ARE SOME OF THE CAUSES OF AUTONOMIC DYSFUNCTION?

The autonomic nervous system may be injured in a variety of ways:

- Head Injury (concussions)
- Emotional Trauma (intense emotional events, emotional concussions)
- Metabolic Injury (medications, chemotherapy or radiation, heat stroke, alcohol intoxication)
- Inflammatory Injury (infections, tobacco smoke, excessive omega-6 fatty acid intake, vaccines, surgery, autoimmunity, allergy tests or allergy shots)
- Intestinal Bacterial Overgrowth (SIBO, dysbiosis)
- Pregnancy

HOW DOES RECOVERY OF AUTONOMIC DYSFUNCTION OCCUR?

I have found that the improvement and recovery of autonomic dysfunction is possible by inducing the nervous system and organs to repair themselves by normalizing inflammation control mechanisms, inducing natural stem cell production, and reactivating innate restorative mechanisms.

I have also found that recovery from autonomic dysfunction is a realistic goal and it may occur decades after the injury and the dysfunction first began.

- Symptoms Lessen as the Brain Repairs
- Core Nutrients Lower Brain Inflammation
- Stem Cell Production Resumes
- Natural Brain Repair Mechanisms Activate
- Vagus Nerve Stimulation Speeds Recovery (Adults)
- Cell Functions Normalize
- Long Term Damage is Reversible

THE FIVE STAGES OF AUTONOMIC DYSFUNCTION

AAutonomic dysfunction occurs when the nerves that carry information from the brain to the heart, bladder, intestines, sweat glands, pupils, and blood vessels no longer function properly.

This improper function may affect different organ systems in different people, so symptoms may vary greatly from one person to the next person.

This improper function may also affect multiple systems within one person at the same time, which accounts for a number of health problems that seem very different and unrelated, but actually originate in this one area of the nervous system.

A patient's timeline of events and illnesses will begin to make sense once they understand that autonomic injury and inflammation causes a variety of symptoms, and then it triggers diseases such as diabetes, cancer, heart failure, and Alzheimer's.

My treatment program, The Nemechek Protocol™ for Autonomic Recovery, puts these pieces together and treats the underlying cause. The first step is spectral analysis of the autonomic nervous system to determine the type and severity of your autonomic dysfunction.

Spectral analysis allows us to detect your sympathetic branch and parasympathetic patterns of damage. There are five stages of autonomic dysfunction that show up as different strengths of sympathetic and parasympathetic functions. Your test results are a biomarker for your brain's overall health and ability to correctly run your body.

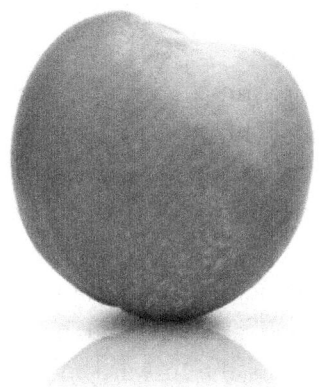

STAGES 1 AND 2

Stage 1 and Stage 2 of autonomic dysfunction do not have noticeable symptoms yet these preclinical changes in brain function are detected during spectral analysis autonomic testing.

Identifying subtle changes in brain functions allows me the opportunity to work with my patients to reverse the damage and to prevent future complications.

As autonomic dysfunction progresses into Stage 3, people become unable to compensate for their autonomic abnormalities and their ability to handle disease and stress becomes impaired.

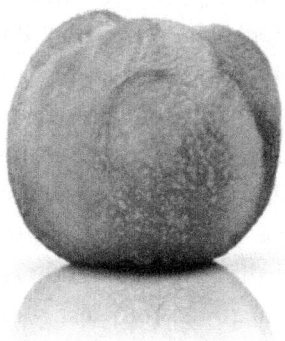

STAGE 3

In Stage 3 of autonomic dysfunction people start to experience symptoms that affect their daily life. At this point, autonomic dysfunction causes people to experience things such as heartburn, headaches, intestinal distress, dizziness, excessive hunger or thirst, anxiety, sexual dysfunction (women and men), or poor sleep.

The progression of autonomic dysfunction also brings the inability to control blood pressure and heart rates (A-fib, flutter, palpitations, POTS), affects the forward movement of the digestive tract, and proper breathing (sleep apnea).

People experience problems with their immune system, hormone levels, and organ functions. People no longer bounce back from illnesses or injury and they may suffer from chronic fatigue or chronic pain.

As autonomic function declines, and inflammation rises, their symptoms may also be mental or emotional in nature. People have a harder time recovering from trauma and they may suffer from anxiety, panic attacks, depression, postpartum depression, and PTSD.

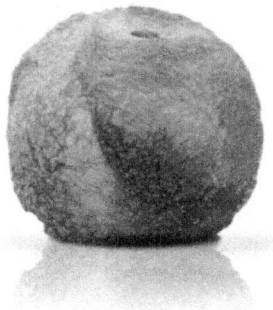

STAGE 4

In Stage 4 of autonomic dysfunction, multiple systems in the body malfunction and people feel increasingly worse. Blood pressure or blood sugars get harder to regulate even with medications, and people have poor responses to other medical therapies.

As their heart, immune system, and hormonal systems malfunction, and as their depression or anxiety increases, people turn to a variety of medical specialties searching for answers and diagnoses to explain their avalanche of brain and body dysfunction.

Worsening autonomic patterns of sympathetic and/or parasympathetic weakness at rest, also called Low Heart Rate Variability (low HRV) or Advanced Autonomic Dysfunction, disrupts their daily quality of life. Low HRV leaves them at a higher risk of death from all causes because their body is unable to respond to things like pneumonia, cancer, and infections.

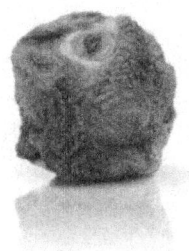

STAGE 5

Like Stages 1 and 2, the decline into Stage 5 of autonomic dysfunction may be silent but it is detected through autonomic spectral analysis. As the autonomics continue to malfunction, autonomic testing reveals weaker parasympathetic functions and increased Low HRV (Heart Rate Variability).

The most advanced autonomic test patterns of weak parasympathetic functions are Diabetic Autonomic Neuropathy (DAN), and then Cardiac Autonomic Neuropathy (CAN), which has a 50% mortality rate within five years if left untreated.

The autonomics are so suppressed in Stage 5 that the person experiences more difficulties at times, such as, when they are artificially asleep under anesthesia, maintaining proper control of their heart rhythms which increases their risk of sudden cardiac death.

One of the most important things I have discovered is that all five stages of autonomic dysfunction are capable of improvement or repair, even decades after the autonomic injury. For 30 years, I have been willing to adopt and adapt any treatment approach that offers a chance to improve the health and well being of my patients.

I am fortunate that my education and experience with complex diseases allows me to significantly impact peoples' lives. I am proud to say I have developed The Nemechek Protocol™ for Autonomic

Recovery that has improved the health of many, even after they had been told there were no other options available.

Karla and Her Headaches

Karla is a 42-year-old woman who was suffering from headaches that occurred almost daily, but once or twice per week would become so severe they were incapacitating. Her headaches seemed to begin shortly after waking and would worsen through the day. She noticed her headaches would worsen when she was sitting still while riding in a car or while on an airplane. Before menstruation her headaches almost always increased in intensity and were often accompanied with anxiety, fatigue, brain fog, tightness of the neck and shoulders, and occasional numbness of the hands.

She had always had occasional mild headaches but they increased in intensity after having her gall bladder removed. Since then her headaches became much more frequent and severe, and interestingly she now had problems with occasional heartburn from bananas and coffee.

Karla's autonomic testing revealed severe underlying sympathetic weakness (the red bar is below the grey normal range), which makes it hard for the body to pump enough blood upwards into the head and neck region when someone is upright. Sympathetic weakness while standing is often referred to as sympathetic withdrawal.

Sympathetic Weakness or Withdrawal

Karla's neck and scalp pain are referred to as 'coat hanger pain' and they are caused by an inadequate delivery of oxygen into the muscles of the neck and scalp.

Low blood pressure into the head and neck can also cause fatigue, poor cognition (i.e. brain fog, ADD, ADHD), anxiety, numbness of hands, face or neck (i.e. neuronal ischemia), fidgety behaviors (toe tapping, sitting cross legged or with a leg folded underneath, frequent changing of body position while seated), and symptoms commonly misunderstood to be from "low blood sugar".

These low blood pressure symptoms often begin after getting out of bed and they worsen through the day. Sitting or standing still, becoming overheated, decreases in progesterone levels (pre-menstruation or menopause), and mild viral infections may all exacerbate the low blood pressure and symptoms.

Karla's previous mild headaches worsened after her gall bladder surgery because the stress of the surgery caused an inflammatory injury to her autonomic nervous system, and it also triggered bacterial overgrowth of the small intestine, which caused her intestinal problems.

Karla had seen several health providers but her tests always came up normal, and she walked away with a few prescriptions that were just meant to cover up her symptoms. She was frustrated because no one seemed to be trying to find and fix the source of her problems.

Within two months of starting The Nemechek Protocol™ for Autonomic Recovery, Karla's headaches had dramatically decreased in frequency and intensity, as had most of her other symptoms.

The intestinal issues almost completely resolved within the first two weeks of treatment.

After six months Karla's autonomic testing revealed her sympathetic weakness had returned to normal.

Normalized Sympathetic Function

She has not had a headache within the last three months, and she only needs to take a simple and inexpensive regimen of supplements that she can buy from a variety of online retailers.

Her anxieties, fatigue, brain fog, tightness of the neck and shoulders, and numbness of the hands have all resolved as well.

3
BACTERIAL OVERGROWTH CONTRIBUTES TO AUTONOMIC DYSFUNCTION

There is growing scientific evidence that an imbalance of intestinal bacteria, along with excessive inflammation within the brain, are responsible for the features associated with migraine headaches, heartburn, IBS, "brain fog", lightheadedness or dizziness, chronic fatigue, generalized anxiety, obesity, chronic depression, and PTSD.

In children, imbalances of intestinal bacteria and inflammation are major factors in the development of autism, ADD/ADHD, mood disorders, and developmental delay.

This imbalance of intestinal bacteria also contributes to worsening autonomic nervous system dysfunction. To begin to understand the connection between our intestinal bacteria and our autonomics, we must start at the beginning, with our development as children.

NORMAL BRAIN DEVELOPMENT

Normal brain development requires a healthy environment for the brain to develop fully and quickly. A child is born with approximately

100 billion neurons and they must trim these down to 50 billion neurons by the time they are 18 years old.

Failure to trim the neurons fast enough may lead to developmental issues. If the failure to trim is mild and the neurons simply are not being trimmed fast enough, we often refer to this as developmental delay. If the neuronal trimming process has severely slowed or even stopped completely, the child may be classified as having mental retardation.

The common cause of altered neuronal pruning is from impaired functioning of a specialized central nervous system white blood cell known as microglia.

Microglia are often referred to as the 'master gardener' because one of their primary roles is to tend to the neurons that branch throughout the brain, like the branches of plants throughout a garden.

Microglia tend to the neuron branches by either pruning them to get rid of them, or by protecting and repairing them.

The development and distribution of neurons is felt to be somewhat random, as the child's brain has to discover a connection between bodily movements and brain functions.

The development process involves forming the pathways that will allow your child to track your face with their eyes, or roll over in their crib. These behaviors occur only when the child's brain finds the neurons that connect the thought (follow mothers face) to the action (move my eyes and head).

Microglia sense these neuronal pathways are important and start nurturing and protecting them. If other neurons are not being used in any meaningful way, they will eventually be trimmed away as excess.

The process, of pruning away the excessive neurons, is necessary for the brain to survive. Neurons consume large amounts of energy, and it is inefficient for the human body to spend energy on pathways that are not important for survival.

At the time of birth the brain consumes nearly 85% of all oxygen and calories, whereas by the age of 18 years this is "pruned down" and then it only consumes 20%. From an evolutionary viewpoint, this is a much more manageable percentage.

The neuronal pruning process continues throughout the child's life as they learn to crawl, stand upright, talk, walk, run, read, calculate, and mature into young adults.

The microglia not only trim and maintain the normal sequence of maturation, they also help repair the brain injuries that can occur from physical (concussion and sub-concussive injuries), emotional (bullying, intense fear), and inflammatory (surgery, fractures, vaccinations) traumas.

Unfortunately, the microglia function can be altered by the leakage of lipopolysaccharide (LPS), which is fragments of bacterial cell membranes that are leaked into the blood stream when bacterial overgrowth of the small intestine occurs.

The microglia, altered by LPS, are referred to as primed microglia.

MICROGLIA AND ABNORMAL BRAIN DEVELOPMENT

In the womb, a child's intestinal tract contains no bacteria. It is only after a child is born that a child's intestinal tract becomes colonized with their mother's blend of bacteria.

Regardless whether the birth is vaginal or by caesarian section, the child's intestinal bacterial blend matches the bacterial blend of the mother. If the mother's bacterial blend is off a bit then the child's bacterial blend is off a bit as well.

But the bacterial issue is not just a mother-child issue; both parents contribute in different ways. The genes contributed by the mother or the father can determine which bacteria will overgrow, or what those bacteria might do once they overgrow. It is a complex combination of the mother's bacterial blend that may malfunction according to the father's genetic instructions.

Many, if not most, individuals have abnormal blends of intestinal bacteria to some degree. If the child's newly colonized intestinal bacterial is out of balance, bacterial overgrowth (SIBO) may occur shortly after birth and, depending on the severity of the bacterial overgrowth, the impairment of microglial pruning may begin shortly after birth.

In other children, their bacterial blend may only be mildly imbalanced and incapable of triggering impairment of the microglia pruning process. Their bacterial blend may require an additional push from a round of antibiotics, antacids, surgery, or a vaccination.

A SIMPLE DESCRIPTION OF BACTERIAL OVERGROWTH

Bacterial overgrowth is a condition where the child's own bacteria, which should only reside at the bottom of their colon, have replicated and migrated up into the child's small intestine.

This is a massive disruption for the normally balanced intestinal bacterial system. Bacteria from the colon are very different from the bacteria that live in the small intestine. The two types of bacteria are so different that I explain to my patients that one type is like birds (the normal residents of the small intestine) and the other type is like fish (the normal residents of the colon). The acidity of their respective environments, and the motility of the intestinal tract, seem to be the main reasons that these two types of bacteria remain separated.

The small intestine is a relatively acidic environment whereas the colon (large intestine) is much more alkaline.

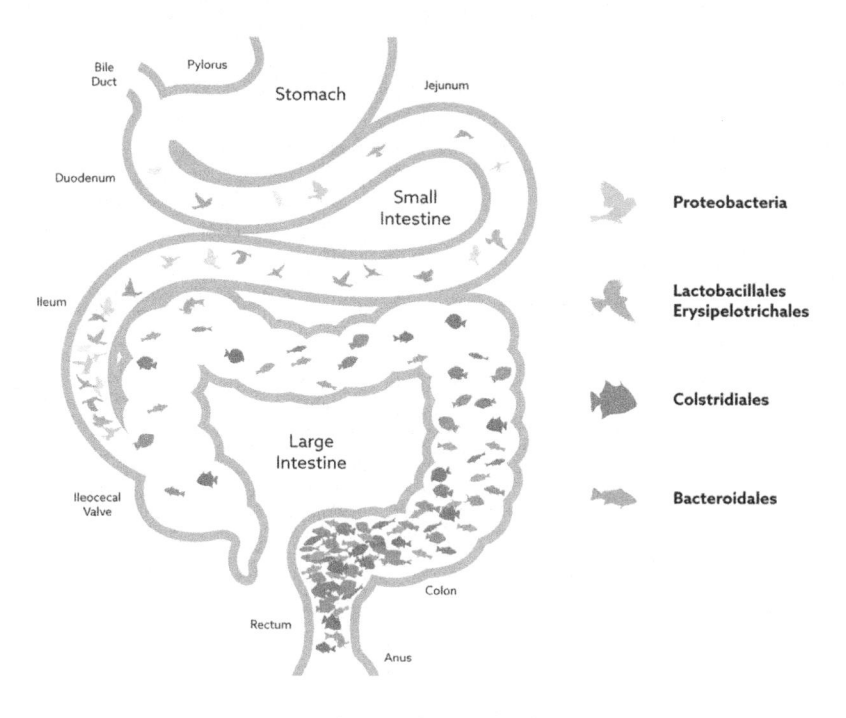

Normal Intestinal Bacterial Balance

Furthermore, there is a very large difference in the concentration of the bacteria. For every individual "bird" bacterium in the upper small intestine, there is normally a hundred million "fish" bacteria living in the lowest portion of the colon. That is an enormous difference. Bacterial overgrowth occurs when the "fish" bacteria migrate up into the small intestinal tract and start living up with the "birds". Everyone understands that fish should not be living up with birds.

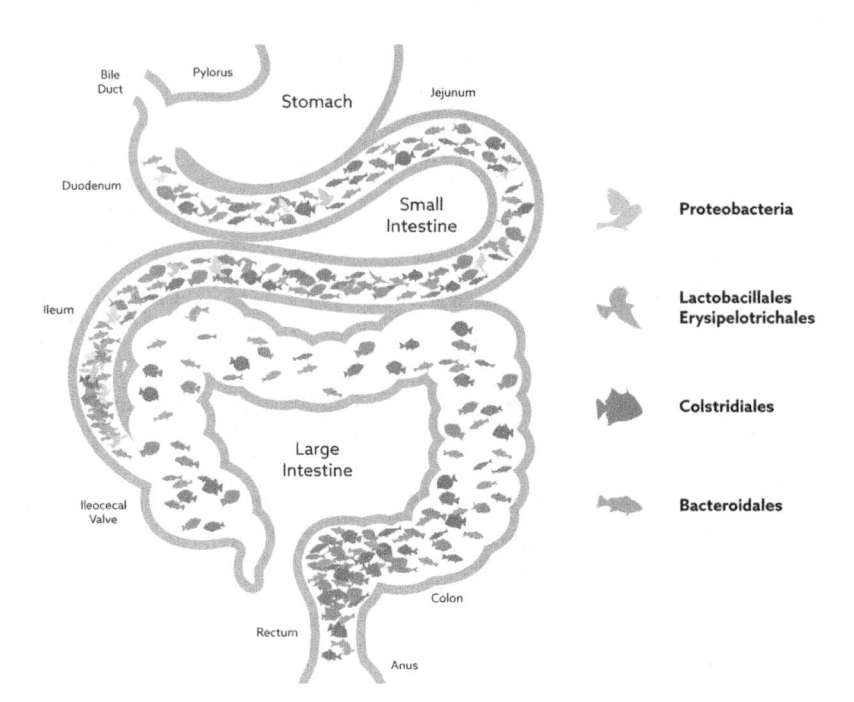

Bacterial Overgrowth of the Small Intestine

After they have migrated into the small intestine, colonic bacteria can create inflammation, influence cell behavior, produce acid, emit toxins and gases, get excited or react to different foods (tomatoes, bananas, milk, citrus, etc.), cause skin disruptions (eczema, hives, rashes), and send signals to the brain through the autonomic nervous system that disrupts the brain, body, and cell functions.

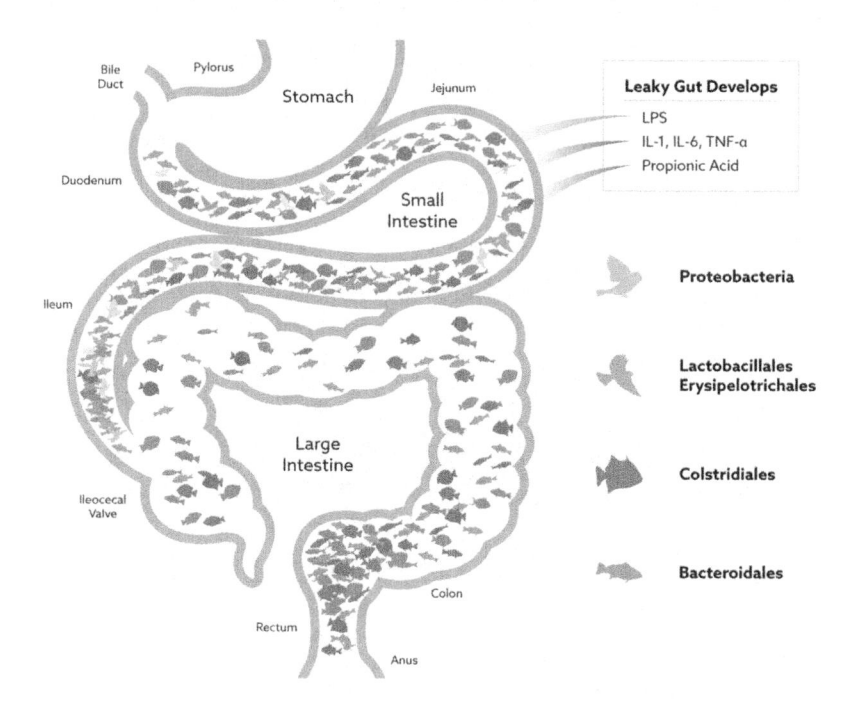

When bacterial overgrowth occurs fragments of bacteria cell membrane called lipopolysaccharide (LPS) leak into the blood stream and flow into the brain where the LPS alters the function of a special white blood cell known as microglia.

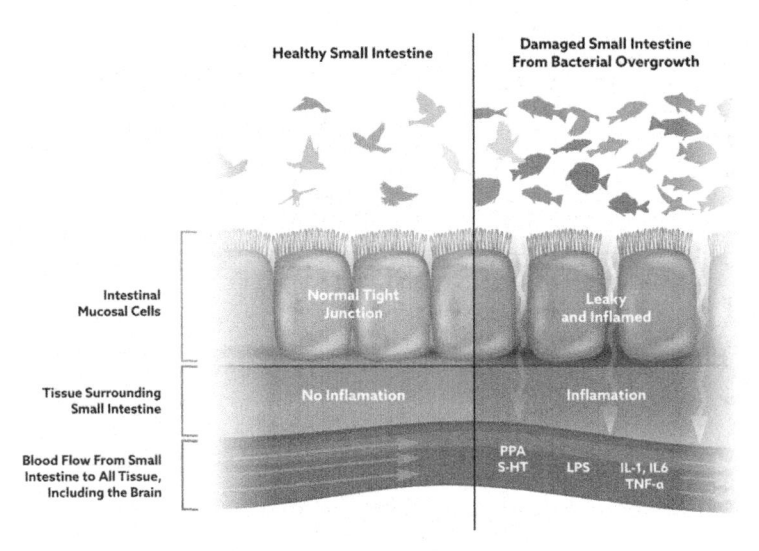

Healthy Small Intestine | **Damaged Small Intestine From Bacterial Overgrowth**

- Intestinal Mucosal Cells
- Normal Tight Junction | Leaky and Inflamed
- Tissue Surrounding Small Intestine
- No Inflamation | Inflamation
- Blood Flow From Small Intestine to All Tissue, Including the Brain
- PPA S-HT | LPS   IL-1, IL6 TNF-α

PPA: Propionic Acid   S-HT: Serotonin   LPS: Lipopolysaccharide   IL-1, IL-6, TNF-α: Inflammatory Cytokines

We call these altered microglia "primed microglia" and their function changes from a helpful cell that repairs damaged neurons, into an unhealthy cell that prevents normal development.

Overgrowth → LPS leakage → Primed Microglia

The bacterial overgrowth and LPS seepage to the brain often happens at the time of birth and worsens later in life as we experience other events that worsen bacterial overgrowth, such as antibiotics, anesthesia, abdominal surgeries, colonoscopies, and any form of brain injury.

The bacterial overgrowth of the small intestine interferes with brain repair because the microglia are no longer in a repair mode, instead the primed microglia have switched into a damage-causing mode.

Bacterial Overgrowth and Microglia Recap:

- Helpful, normal microglia help us develop normally during childhood.
- Colonic bacteria (fish) are migrating too high into the small intestine (birds).
- Bacterial overgrowth = when colonic bacteria (fish) are living up with the small intestine bacteria (birds).
- Bacterial overgrowth causes LPS leakage, which changes cell function to "Primed Microglia"
- Primed microglia are no longer helpful, primed microglia are harmful.
- Primed microglia do not perform normal neuron pruning in children or repair brain injuries in adults or children.

PRIMED MICROGLIA MAGNIFY DAMAGE AND LIMIT RECOVERY

Primed microglia will also worsen the degree of damage caused by the injury and prevent stem cells and other repair mechanisms from fully repairing the brain damage that would have fully recovered in an otherwise healthy brain, with normally functioning microglia.

Figure

Pruning and Repairing Microglia → "Priming" Triggered by LPS → **Pro-Inflammatory M1 - Microglia**

IL-1, IL6, TNF-α   LPS   IL-1, IL6, TNF-α

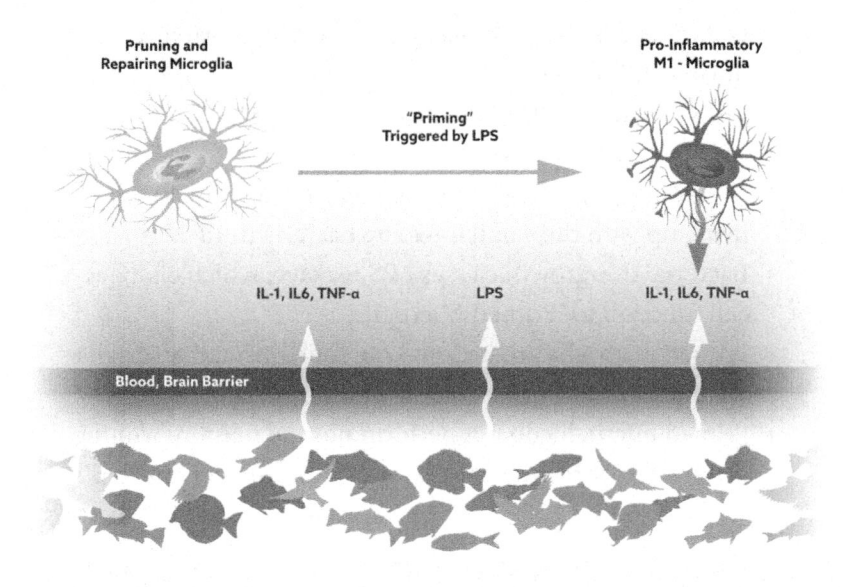

Blood, Brain Barrier

PPA: Propionic Acid   S-HT: Serotonin   LPS: Lipopolysaccharide   IL-1, IL-6, TNF-α: Inflammatory Cytokines

The impairment of microglia may also be responsible for the abnormal white matter structure within the brain that seems to be associated with sensory perception disorders.

More damage and less recovery are the hallmark features of a pathological process called cumulative brain injury or CBI.

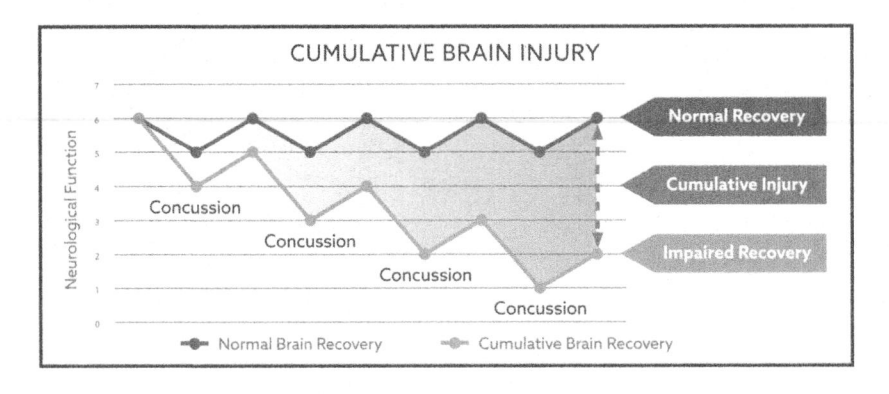

CUMULATIVE BRAIN INJURY

(Neurological Function vs. Concussions; Normal Recovery, Cumulative Injury, Impaired Recovery)

— Normal Brain Recovery   — Cumulative Brain Recovery

Cumulative brain injury from primed microglia is occurring at an epidemic rate throughout the population, and is the predominant feature behind the well-publicized problems of professional football players contracting chronic traumatic encephalopathy (CTE). Cumulative brain injury develops not only from physical injuries but can occur from emotional and inflammatory (surgery, fractures, vaccines) injuries as well.

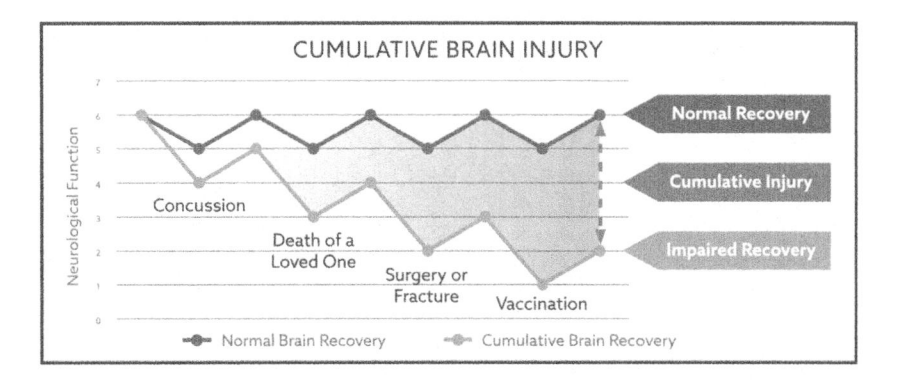

CUMULATIVE BRAIN INJURY

Chart showing Neurological Function over time with events: Concussion, Death of a Loved One, Surgery or Fracture, Vaccination. Lines indicate Normal Brain Recovery vs Cumulative Brain Recovery, with labels Normal Recovery, Cumulative Injury, and Impaired Recovery.

In addition to primed microglia not pruning correctly and causing varying degrees of developmental delay, the cumulative brain injury effect from primed microglia is also allowing small brain injuries to stack upon previously unresolved brain injuries.

The process of cumulative brain injuries, due to bacterial overgrowth and primed microglia, is one of the most common mechanisms by which a person's autonomic nervous system becomes damaged throughout their life. When brain injuries are not repaired they impact on how the brain is able to work, and control the body, through the autonomic nervous system.

Cumulative damage thus results in a variety of symptoms and in conditions such as migraine headaches, heartburn, IBS, increased cravings for salt or sugar, chronic fatigue, frequent urination, chronic neck pain, memory problems, constipation, erectile dysfunction, premenstrual syndrome, attention deficit disorder (ADD), hyperactivity, headaches, anxiety, and chronic depression.

4
TAKE THE AUTONOMIC BRAIN QUIZ

THE AUTONOMIC BRAIN QUIZ

Studies indicate that 80% of chronic disease is caused by dysfunction of the autonomic nervous system. Autonomic dysfunction impairs the normal function of all organs (kidneys, liver, heart, circulation, intestines, and bladder), the immune system, hormone production, and your emotional balance.

Many common but disturbing symptoms are a sign of a larger problem, of autonomic dysfunction. Many medical conditions such as diabetes, high blood pressure, gout, sleep apnea, chronic headaches or migraines, chronic fatigue, heart rhythm problems, heartburn, and chronic constipation have autonomic dysfunction as a central mechanism in their development.

Fortunately, there is a simple and painless autonomic test called spectral analysis that accurately measures the health of your autonomic nervous system. If abnormalities are detected, new techniques have been developed to help the autonomic nervous system to recover.

Recovery and normalization of autonomic function often leads to a remarkable improvement and even complete reversal of the medical conditions listed above.

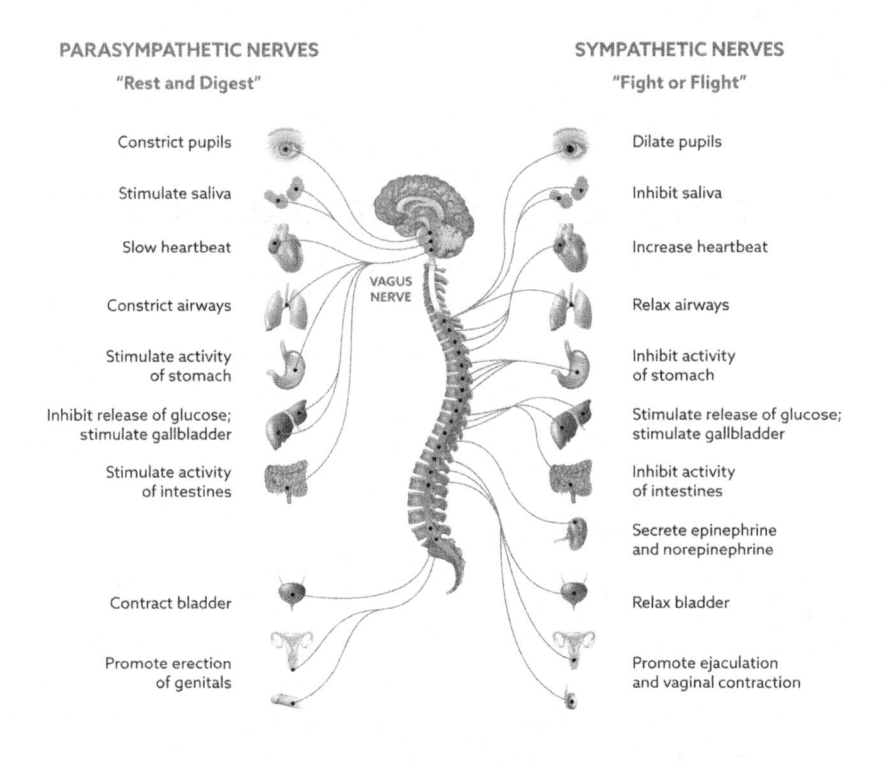

PARASYMPATHETIC NERVES "Rest and Digest"	SYMPATHETIC NERVES "Fight or Flight"
Constrict pupils	Dilate pupils
Stimulate saliva	Inhibit saliva
Slow heartbeat	Increase heartbeat
Constrict airways	Relax airways
Stimulate activity of stomach	Inhibit activity of stomach
Inhibit release of glucose; stimulate gallbladder	Stimulate release of glucose; stimulate gallbladder
Stimulate activity of intestines	Inhibit activity of intestines
	Secrete epinephrine and norepinephrine
Contract bladder	Relax bladder
Promote erection of genitals	Promote ejaculation and vaginal contraction

The Autonomic Nervous System

If your symptoms have lasted for more than three months you may be developing chronic autonomic damage from cumulative brain injury.

IF YOU CHECK MORE THAN 3 BOXES YOU MAY HAVE AUTONOMIC DYSFUNCTION

Check the boxes that apply to you.

___ I am occasionally nauseated in the A.M.

___ I am dizzy or lightheaded at times.
___ I frequently feel anxious.
___ I have trouble with memory or concentration.
___ I feel unusually tired during the day.
___ I have "brain fog" at times.
___ I have trouble waking up in the morning.
___ I get frequent headaches or migraines.
___ I feel tightness in my neck or shoulder muscles.
___ I feel thirsty or hungry through the day.
___ My hands, face, or neck go numb periodically.
___ I find myself craving salt or sugar.
___ I become sleepy after a meal.
___ I frequently urinate.
___ I get heartburn or reflux.
___ I experience "PMS" before menstruation.
___ I have trouble sleeping.
___ I have difficulty getting an erection.
___ I have trouble seeing in bright or dim light.
___ I have passed out or fainted.
___ I feel weak when I get hot.
___ I have heart palpitations or an abnormal rhythm.
___ I feel excessively hot or cold.
___ My labs are fine but I feel "off".

Checking "yes" to the common symptoms of autonomic dysfunction may help you realize that the various symptoms represented in those boxes actually share common causes within the nervous system.

Autonomic testing via spectral analysis is a painless and rapid 17-minute test and provides critical information as to why you do not feel well. This may be the first diagnostic step towards understanding the underlying problem and in knowing how to make you feel healthy again.

Next, think about events in your life that may have caused autonomic dysfunction. Keep in mind that brain and nervous system injuries do not always require a significant physical event such as a severe concussion or blacking out.

Your autonomic dysfunction may also have been caused by medications used in general anesthesia, an imbalance of intestinal bacteria, pregnancy, mild concussions, emotionally traumatic events, an imbalance of dietary omega-6 and omega-3 fatty acid intake, and by processed foods.

5

AUTONOMIC TESTING VIA SPECTRAL ANALYSIS

The electrical fluctuation noted on a 3-lead electrocardiogram signal is a combination of the electrical depolarization of heart muscle during contraction as well as the signaling from the autonomic nervous system.

These different signals are blended together in a manner similar to the variety of signals coming to one's home from a cable or Internet service. In the home, the signal is put into a cable box that separates the signals into a variety of different television channels, for instance.

In a similar fashion, spectral analysis takes the single electrical impulse from the electrocardiogram and separates the cardiac and autonomic signals using their unique individual frequencies.

Spectral analysis is the only method that obtains direct measurements of both autonomic branches simultaneously, in a scientifically valid, non-invasive manner.

Concussions may result in damage to many portions of the central nervous system but it is the damage to the autonomic nervous system that causes the most physically disabling symptoms.

Headaches, fatigue, poor cognition, altered vision, and altered balance are often simply reflections of impaired blood pressure and oxygen delivery to the brain.

Prior testing is not necessary to determine if underlying autonomic damage exists. Any variation from the well-defined normal responses (based on age and gender) is scientifically valid evidence of autonomic damage.

The measurement of autonomic function via spectral analysis has been utilized in almost 3,000 different research publications.

A complete spectral analysis tests requires only 17 minutes and provides precise autonomic measurement. It is one of the few methodologies that can directly measure of autonomic signaling from brain to heart.

Other common forms of autonomic testing such as tilt table testing, memory tests, sudomotor tests, visual evoked potentials, and physical examination features either do not *directly* measure the autonomic function but rather *infer* functionality from physical changes, may be prone to performance bias, or are not practical for repeat testing because of their expense or the lack of portability of the testing equipment.

Spectral analysis utilizing the ANSAR ANX 3.0 software utilizes 4 autonomic testing maneuvers known as Resting Baseline Test, Deep Breathing, Valsalva Maneuver and the 5-Minute Stand. Each testing component provides a different view of autonomic functioning.

The first testing component, the Resting Baseline Test involves having the subject sit quietly for 5 minutes while measuring sympathetic and parasympathetic electrical activity, blood pressure, and pulse. This gives a good measure of resting sympathovagal tone and overall autonomic health.

	Interpretation	VALUE	NORMAL RANGE
Mean Heart Rate	Normal	66 bpm	
Range Heart Rate (Range HR, Max - Min)	Normal	37 bpm	
Sympathetic Modulation (LFa)	Normal	5.14 bpm²	
Parasympathetic Modulation (HFa)	Normal	8.81 bpm²	
Sympathovagal Balance (LFa/HFa)	Low Normal	0.58	
Systolic Blood Pressure	Elevated	120 mmHg	
Diastolic Blood Pressure		79 mmHg	

Resting Baseline Test

Damage noted in the Resting Baseline Test often can demonstrate weaknesses of both parasympathetic and sympathetic functioning, known as low heart rate variability (HRV).

Low HRV is associated with an increased risk of death from all causes because the brain is unable to command the body to respond correctly to stressors such as injury, pneumonia, heart attacks, or cancer.

The Resting Baseline Test may also detect Cardiac Autonomic Neuropathy, a state of extreme sympathovagal imbalance that is associated with increased risk from cardiac arrest.

It may also detect Elevated HRV, the underlying phenomena responsible for cardiac arrhythmias such as atrial fibrillation and atrial flutter.

The second testing component is Deep Breathing and involves the slowed controlled inhalation and exhalation of 6 breaths over a 1 minute time frame.

This tests for the ability of the brain to increase parasympathetic drive while under stress.

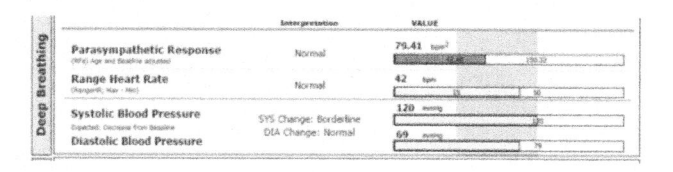

	Interpretation	VALUE	
Parasympathetic Response (RFa) Age and Baseline adjusted	Normal	79.41 bpm²	
Range Heart Rate (Range HR, Max - Min)	Normal	42 bpm	
Systolic Blood Pressure	SYS Change: Borderline	120 mmHg	
Diastolic Blood Pressure	DIA Change: Normal	69 mmHg	

Paced Breathing

Damage here is reflected as a weakness in parasympathetic signaling and results in increased inflammation in the brain, joints, or tissues, and the worsening of autoimmune disorders.

The increased inflammatory state is critical in concussion recovery, because increased inflammatory cytokines within the central nervous system is a major factor preventing recovery from concussions, depression, and PTSD.

Impaired parasympathetic functioning also contributes to heartburn, constipation, bloating and cramping, and leads to abnormal hormone regulation.

The third and fourth components, the Valsalva Maneuver and the 5-Minute Stand test, measure both sympathetic and parasympathetic functioning simultaneously.

Valsalva Maneuver

These tests shift the burden of maintaining proper brain blood pressure and oxygen delivery to the sympathetic branch, requiring a simultaneous, and balanced, increase in sympathetic activation with a decrease in parasympathetic activation.

5-Minute Stand Test

Excessive parasympathetic activation on either of these tests is known as Paradoxical Parasympathetic Syndrome and leads to the development of poor exercise recovery, sleep apnea, restless leg syndrome, non-restorative sleep, headaches, erectile dysfunction, bladder dysfunction, and hot flashes.

A weak sympathetic response is referred to as Sympathetic Withdrawal and leads to the development of poor focus, memory and concentration, impaired vision in dim light, altered balance, anxiousness, fatigue, headaches, neck tightness, hand numbness, and increased thirst.

Sympathetic Withdrawal also causes increased hunger leading to obesity, and an increase in the subsequent risk of developing diabetes, cancer, heart disease, heart failure, clotting disorders, macular degeneration, ALS, Alzheimer's and Parkinson's disease.

Collectively, these four tests provide a rapid and easily repeatable method to assess recovery from traumatic brain injury, and to assess and design treatment regimens that can accelerate autonomic recovery.

6
RECOVERY OF POST CONCUSSION SYNDROME IN A YOUNG ATHLETE

This example involves a 16-year old male who is participating at an extremely advanced level of soccer.

He was experiencing difficulty with concentration and mental focus at times, which was not only affecting his school work, but also his decision making on the soccer field.

Although he had been hit in the head a few times while playing, both the patient and his mother could not recall any specific injury that stood out as a concussion-inducing event.

What is not well appreciated in the field of concussion management is that if an individual's repair process is not operating correctly, a multitude of relatively minor head traumas will not be repaired and trauma will accumulate, one on top of another.

Given enough occurrences, this process of accumulated damage on prior damage has the cumulative effect of a single significant injury.

Spectral analysis testing on this young man revealed the common finding of impaired sympathetic response on the 5-Minute Stand Test referred to as Sympathetic Withdrawal.

5-Minute Stand Test

The patient was started on The Nemechek ProtocolTM for Autonomic Recovery (Pat. Pending), a personalized recovery program balancing his dietary omega fatty acids intake and treatment of bacterial translocation of LPS.

He was also started on Vagus neuromodulation (Vagus nerve stimulation) to help augment inflammation control via the cholinergic anti-inflammatory pathway.

Paced Breathing

Within 3 months the patient's autonomic function had completely normalized and his difficulty with mental focus and concentration had completely normalized.

7

AUTONOMIC RECOVERY FROM A HEAD INJURY OCCURRING 30-YEARS PRIOR

This example involves a male patient who experienced a severe concussion in 1978 while playing football at the age of 18.

With the relative lack of medical understanding about traumatic brain injuries and concussion at the time, there was no medical follow-up and the patient enrolled into college.

The patient is now a 55-year old professional and recalls how his ability to focus and memorize material during college was greatly reduced compared to his ability while in high school. It was not until later in his life that he realized his concussion had severely affected his cognition to such an extent that he has little, to no, memory of many aspects of his time during college. He cannot even remember any details regarding the apartment he lived in for the last three years of school.

Throughout his adult life he had great difficulty remembering numbers and names and developed a process of written notes, reminders, and reading techniques to help him excel in his career as a physician. He also experienced episodes of unexplained fatigue and anxiousness.

He underwent autonomic testing in 2011 and it revealed a weak sympathetic response on the Stand Test, a condition known as Sympathetic Withdrawal.

As has been discussed previously, Sympathetic Withdrawal results in the inadequate delivery of oxygen into the brain and this was the major cause of this patient's cognitive, anxiety, and fatigue issues.

		Interpretation	VALUE
Stand	**Mean Heart Rate** Expected: >10% but <30 beats increase from Baseline	Normal	91 bpm 91.30 113.00
	Range Heart Rate (RangeHR; Max - Min)	Normal	20 bpm 15 50
	Sympathetic Response (LPa) Expected: 20% - 400% increase from Baseline	Low	1.67 bpm² 4.34 20.57
	Parasympathetic Response (RPa) Expected: Decrease from Baseline	Normal	0.36 bpm² 1.62
	Systolic Blood Pressure Expected: Up to 20 mmHg increase from Baseline	SYS Change: Borderline Low DIA Change: Normal	133 mmHg 116 166
	Diastolic Blood Pressure Expected: 10 mmHg decrease to 15 mmHg increase from Baseline		91 mmHg 80 105

5-Minute Stand Test

The Deep Breathing portion of the test also showed damage to the parasympathetic branch of his autonomic nervous system. The brain controls inflammation via the parasympathetic branch and this damage commonly results in an elevated inflammatory state within the body as well as the brain. The parasympathetic damage certainly contributed to his lack of recovery from the concussion as well as his recurrent back and shoulder inflammatory pain from past injuries.

		Interpretation	VALUE
Deep Breathing	**Parasympathetic Response** (RPa) Age and Baseline adjusted	Borderline Low	22.01 bpm¹ 70 91.11
	Range Heart Rate (RangeHR; Max - Min)	Normal	21 bpm 15 50
	Systolic Blood Pressure Expected: Decrease from Baseline	SYS Change: Borderline DIA Change: Normal	126 mmHg 129
	Diastolic Blood Pressure		72 mmHg 81

Paced Breathing

This patient was started on The Nemechek ProtocolTM for Autonomic Recovery (Pat. Pending) to normalize primed-microglia functions and reduce a wide variety of sources of pro-inflammatory cytokines that contributes to neuroinflammation.

The successful reduction of neuroinflammation must address:

- Linoleic Fatty Acid Neurotoxicity
- Omega-3 Fatty Acid Deficiencies
- Cholinergic Anti-inflammatory Pathway Disruption
- HGMB1 Stimulation
- Neuronal Glycated Protein Accumulation
- Endoplasmic Reticular Stress
- Mitochondrial Oxidative Stress
- Autoimmune Inflammatory Processes
- Chronic Infections (viral, dental, intestinal)
- Tobacco Smoke Exposure

Over the course of 8 months his sympathetic functioning greatly improved and resulted in improvement to his memory, focus, energy levels and anxiousness.

He lost approximately 60 lbs. with his new dietary regimen, and reduced appetite, and his intra-abdominal fat disappeared.

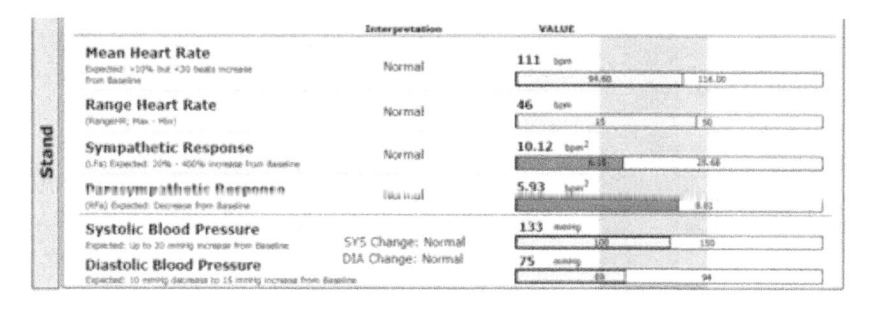

	Interpretation	VALUE
Mean Heart Rate	Normal	111 bpm (94.60 – 114.00)
Range Heart Rate	Normal	46 bpm (15 – 50)
Sympathetic Response	Normal	10.12 bpm² (6.38 – 25.68)
Parasympathetic Response	Normal	5.93 bpm² (8.81)
Systolic Blood Pressure	SYS Change: Normal	133 mmHg (108 – 150)
Diastolic Blood Pressure	DIA Change: Normal	75 mmHg (69 – 94)

5-Minute Stand Test

Likewise, he experienced improvement in parasympathetic function, which along with the dietary changes helped to normalize inflammation control, and resulted in his chronic back and shoulder pain finally stopping after many years.

44 | A SIMPLIFIED GUIDE TO AUTONOMIC DYSFUNCTION

	Interpretation	Value
Parasympathetic Response (RSA) Age and Baseline adjusted	Normal	79.41 bpm² / 150.32
Range Heart Rate (Range@R; Max - Min)	Normal	42 bpm / 15 – 50
Systolic Blood Pressure Expected: Decrease from baseline	SYS Change: Borderline	120 mmHg / 120
Diastolic Blood Pressure	DIA Change: Normal	69 mmHg / 79

Deep Breathing

Paced Breathing

He continues on a regular maintenance dietary program and regular use of the transcutaneous vagus nerve stimulation.

His believes his cognitive functioning is better than it has been in his entire adult life.

8
REVERSAL OF LOW HRV AND CARDIAC AUTONOMIC NEROPATHY

This example involves a 67-year-old female with a history of Diabetes Mellitus Type 2 (adult onset), mild hypertension (high blood pressure), lightheadedness, and migraine headaches.

She had experienced mild headaches and occasional lightheadedness for almost 25 years since she experienced menopause.

The diabetes and hypertension had been slowly worsening over the past 15 years but they became much worse a few months after her husband suddenly passed away from cancer.

Since her husband's death she had gained 55 pounds, felt constantly tired and anxious, and her blood pressure and blood sugars became much more difficult to control.

Her autonomic testing revealed a very dangerous autonomic condition called Cardiac Autonomic Neuropathy or CAN (defined as parasympathetic modulation less than 0.11, plus Sympathovagal Balance greater than 3.0).

	Interpretation	VALUE	NORMAL RANGE
Mean Heart Rate	Normal	66 bpm	60 — 100
Range Heart Rate (RangeHR; Max - Min)	Low	8 bpm	10 — 50
Sympathetic Modulation (LFa)	Low	0.36 bpm^2	0.5 — 10
Parasympathetic Modulation (RFa)	Critically Low	0.04 bpm^2	0.5 — 10
Sympathovagal Balance (LFa/RFa)	High (Indicates a resting Sympathetic excess)	9.72	0.4 — 3
Systolic Blood Pressure	High (Stage 2 Hypertension)	180 mmHg	90 — 120
Diastolic Blood Pressure		95 mmHg	— 90

Initial Baseline (Resting)

Cardiac Autonomic Neuropathy

Individuals with CAN have a 50% chance of death within 5 years if it is left untreated, and CAN is a common finding and cause of death among diabetics.

Individuals with CAN often die from sudden cardiac death, a condition that results in the individual's heart beat increasing up to 300 beats per minute. At this extreme rate, the heart is unable to pump any blood causing the individual to collapse and die.

CAN is an extreme form of another more common autonomic condition called low heart rate variability or low HRV. Low HRV is associated with an increased risk of medical complications from a variety of common conditions such as pneumonia, hip fracture, heart attack, and stroke. Low HRV also increases the risk of depression, hospitalization, and is associated with more aggressive forms of cancer. Low HRV is also associated with an increased risk of death albeit not as severe as that associated with CAN.

Low HRV is defined as weak autonomic function often measured while sitting quietly. Low HRV can be seen as weak parasympathetic function (HF or RFa) or weak sympathetic function (LF or LFa) or a large value for the ratio between the sympathetic and parasympathetic signals (LF/HF, LFa/RFa).

The patient was started on The Nemechek ProtocolTM for Autonomic Recovery, with a treatment regimen designed to address a variety of her inflammatory and metabolic problems that were impeding normal autonomic recovery.

After five months, her Cardiac Autonomic Neuropathy had completely resolved.

	Interpretation	VALUE	NORMAL RANGE
Mean Heart Rate	Normal	73 bpm	60 – 100
Range Heart Rate (RangeHR; Max - Min)	Normal	11 bpm	10 – 50
Sympathetic Modulation (LFa)	Low	0.26 bpm^2	0.5 – 10
Parasympathetic Modulation (RFa)	Normal	1.63 bpm^2	2.5 – 10
Sympathovagal Balance (LFa/RFa)	Low (Indicates a resting Parasympathetic excess)	0.16	0.4 – 3
Systolic Blood Pressure	High (Stage 1 Hypertension)	153 mmHg	90 – 120
Diastolic Blood Pressure		81 mmHg	– 80

Initial Baseline (Resting)

Low HRV (weak sympathetic or LFa strength)

Within seven months her remaining low HRV (notice the weak sympathetic signal in red) had also fully recovered.

	Interpretation	VALUE	NORMAL RANGE
Mean Heart Rate	Normal	65 bpm	60 – 100
Range Heart Rate (RangeHR; Max - Min)	Normal	15 bpm	10 – 50
Sympathetic Modulation (LFa)	Normal	1.16 bpm^2	0.5 – 10
Parasympathetic Modulation (RFa)	Normal	1.40 bpm^2	2.5 – 10
Sympathovagal Balance (LFa/RFa)	Low Normal (CAN risk is minimized)	0.83	0.4 – 3
Systolic Blood Pressure	Normal	116 mmHg	90 – 120
Diastolic Blood Pressure		76 mmHg	– 80

Initial Baseline (Resting)

Normalization of both CAN and Low HRV

She was also able to tolerate a regimen of significant carbohydrate reduction which improved her blood sugar and her blood pressure to the extent that she was able to reduce her dependency on her medications.

9
THE NEMECHEK PROTOCOL™ REVERSES AUTONOMIC DYSFUNCITON

Brain injury can occur from physical, emotional, metabolic, and inflammatory injuries. The injury should be repaired within a few weeks to a few months if normal brain repair mechanisms are functioning.

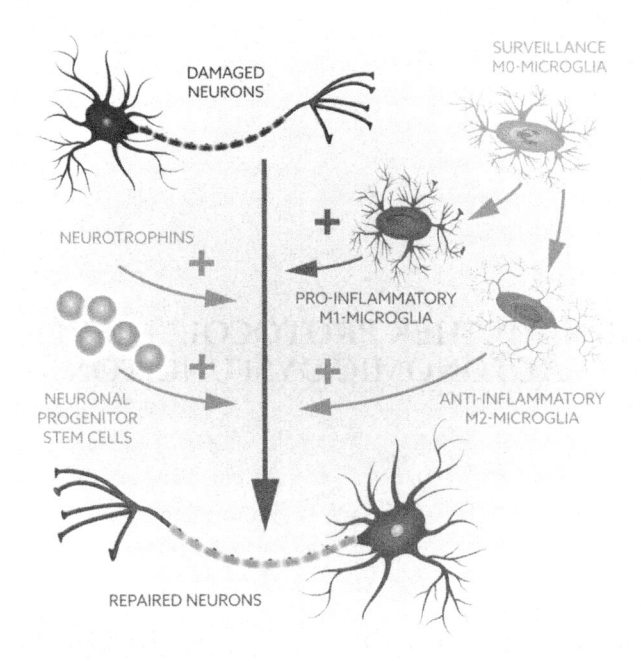

Impairment of the neuron recovery process leads to residual damage due to the combined effect of primed-microglia from bacterial overgrowth which magnifies neuronal damage and excessive pro-inflammatory cytokines.

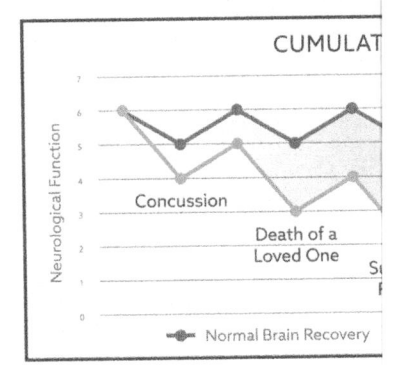

Cumulative brain injury c
lates with each injury, and be
with spectral analysis of the au

The sum effect of VNS u
reversal of symptoms f
chronic depression or PTSD,
generalized anxiety, chronic
(MCI), Alzheimer's dementia,

The Nemechek ProtocolT
chronic medical conditions (P
essential tremor, cancer, card
with microglia dysfunction an

Our book detailing The N
in progress and is expected to

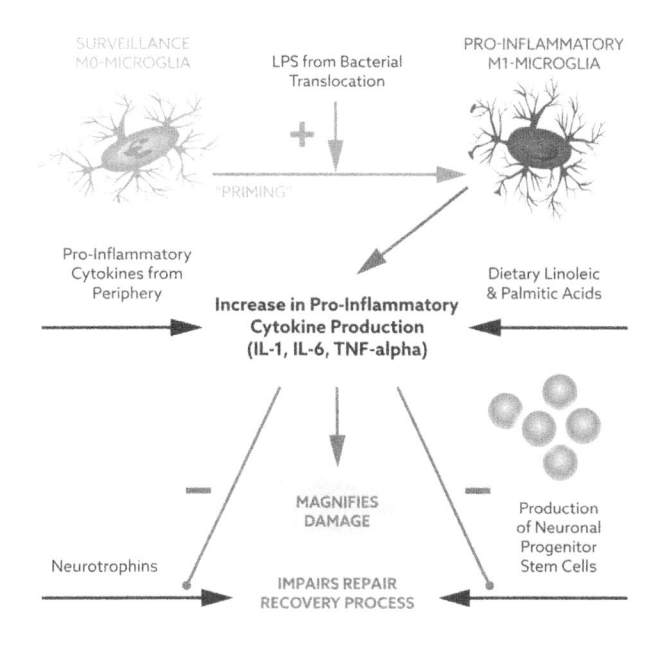

The Nemechek Protocol™ for Autonomic Recovery is a multi-faceted method of treatment that uses a combination of pharmaceutical agents, supplements, vitamins, chemical compounds, dietary restrictions, and neuromodulation of the vagus nerve. The Nemechek Protocol™ reduces the production of pro-inflammatory cytokines from a wide variety of sources that are all capable of affecting the total amount of neuroinflammation within the brain.

SURVEILLANCE
M0-MICROGLIA

"PRIMING"

Rifaximin

Pro-Inflammatory
Cytokines from
Bacterial Overgrowth

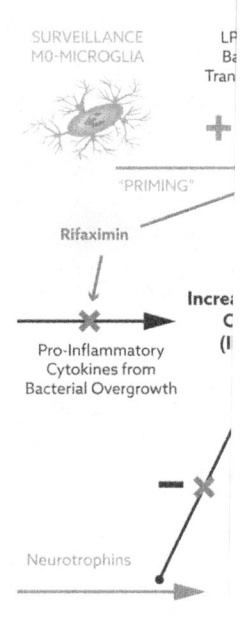

Neurotrophins

The reduction in neuroi
production and functional
natural repair mechanisms

A critical component of
vagus nerve stimulation (V
inflammatory cytokines th
Most importantly, VNS incr
from the M1 inflammatory
phenotype. Primed M1 m
impair recovery resulting ir

SCIENTIFIC REFERENCES

- Wager-Smith, Karen, and Athina Markou. "Depression: A Repair Response to Stress-Induced Neuronal Microdamage That Can Grade into a Chronic Neuroinflammatory Condition?" *Neuroscience and biobehavioral reviews* 35.3 (2011): 742–764.
- Sun, Rao et al. "Hippocampal Activation of Microglia May Underlie the Shared Neurobiology of Comorbid Posttraumatic Stress Disorder and Chronic Pain." *Molecular Pain* 12 (2016): 1744806916679166.
- Goodman, Brent et al. "Autonomic Nervous System Dysfunction in Concussion." Neurology February 12, 2013 vol. 80 no. 7 Supplement P01.265
- La Fountaine, Michael F. et al. "Autonomic Nervous System Responses to Concussion: Arterial Pulse Contour Analysis." *Frontiers in Neurology* 7 (2016): 13.
- Cunningham, Colm. "Microglia and neurodegeneration: the role of systemic inflammation." J Neurosci. 2013 Mar 6;33(10):4216-33.
- Norden, Diana M., Megan M. Muccigrosso, and Jonathan P. Godbout. "Microglial Priming and Enhanced Reactivity

to Secondary Insult in Aging, and Traumatic CNS Injury, and Neurodegenerative Disease." *Neuropharmacology* 96.0 0 (2015): 29–41.
- Calabrese, Francesca et al. "Brain-Derived Neurotrophic Factor: A Bridge between Inflammation and Neuroplasticity." *Frontiers in Cellular Neuroscience* 8 (2014): 430.
- Cunningham, Colm. "Systemic Inflammation and Delirium – Important Co-Factors in the Progression of Dementia." *Biochemical Society transactions* 39.4 (2011): 945–953.
- Goodman et al. "Autonomic Nervous System Dysfunction in Concussion." *Neurology* 80 (1001): P01.265
- McCraty, Rollin, and Fred Shaffer. "Heart Rate Variability: New Perspectives on Physiological Mechanisms, Assessment of Self-Regulatory Capacity, and Health Risk." *Global Advances in Health and Medicine* 4.1 (2015): 46–61. PMC.
- Zhang Q et al. "Activation of the α7 nicotinic receptor promotes lipopolysaccharide-induced conversion of M1 microglia to M2." Am J Transl Res 2017;9(3):971-985.
- Meneses, G. et al. "Electric Stimulation of the Vagus Nerve Reduced Mouse Neuroinflammation Induced by Lipopolysaccharide." *Journal of Inflammation (London, England)* 13 (2016): 33.
- Chang, Philip K-Y et al. "Docosahexaenoic Acid (DHA): A Modulator of Microglia Activity and Dendritic Spine Morphology." *Journal of Neuroinflammation* 12 (2015): 34.
- Harvey, Lloyd D. et al. "Administration of DHA Reduces Endoplasmic Reticulum Stress-Associated Inflammation and Alters Microglial or Macrophage Activation in Traumatic Brain Injury." *ASN NEURO* 7.6 (2015): 1759091415618969.
- Liu, Joanne J. et al. "Pathways of Polyunsaturated Fatty Acid Utilization: Implications for Brain Function in

Neuropsychiatric Health and Disease." *Brain research* 0 (2015): 220–246.
- Gao J et al. "Rifaximin, gut microbes and mucosal inflammation: unraveling a complex relationship." Gut Microbes. 2014 Jul 1;5(4):571-5.
- Nemechek, Patrick and Nemechek, Jean. "Case Study: Reversal of Alzheimer's Dementia with Transcutaneous Vagus Nerve Stimulation (tVNS) in Combination with an Anti-Neuroinflammatory Regimen". International Neuromodulation Society's 13th World Congress, May 2017. Abstract ID: 2718955
- Nemechek, Patrick and Nemechek, Jean. "Reversal of PTSD with Transcutaneous Vagus Nerve Stimulation (tVNS) in Combination with an Anti-Neuroinflammatory Regimen". International Neuromodulation Society's 13th World Congress. May 2017. Abstract ID: 2719545
- Nemechek, Patrick and Nemechek, Jean. "Reversal of Chronic Autonomic Dysfunction with Transcutaneous Vagus Nerve Stimulation (tVNS) as Part of a Multi-Faceted Anti-inflammatory Regimen". International Neuromodulation Society's 13th World Congress. May 2017. Abstract ID: 2719556
- M. S., Borland et al. "Cortical Map Plasticity as a Function of Vagus Nerve Stimulation Intensity." *Brain stimulation* 9.1 (2016): 117–123.
- Plassman BL, Havlik RJ, Steffens DC, Helms MJ, Newman TN, Drosdick D, et al. "Documented head injury in early adulthood and risk of Alzheimer's disease and other dementias." Neurology. 2000; 55:1158–66.
- McKee A and Robinson M. "Military-related traumatic brain injury and neurodegeneration." *Alzheimers Dement.* 2014 June; 10(3 0): S242–S253.
- Gomez-Nicola, Diego, and Delphine Boche. "Post-Mortem Analysis of Neuroinflammatory Changes in Human

Alzheimer's Disease." *Alzheimer's Research & Therapy* 7.1 (2015): 42.
- Eraly, Satish A. et al. "Assessment of Plasma C-Reactive Protein as a Biomarker of PTSD Risk." *JAMA psychiatry* 71.4 (2014): 423–431. *PMC.* Web. 22 Apr. 2017.
- Minassian A et al. "Association of Predeployment Heart Rate Variability With Risk of Postdeployment Posttraumatic Stress Disorder in Active-Duty Marines." JAMA Psychiatry. 2015 Oct;72(10):979-86.

PROJECTS IN DEVELOPMENT

- Fix the Brain, Fix the Body - A Guide for Recovery from Adult Cumulative Brain Injuries with The Nemechek Protocol™
- The Autonomic Advantage™ Brain Injury Recovery Program for Professional and Collegiate Athletic Organizations
- The Nemechek Protocol™ Practitioner Certification Program
- The Autonomic Advantage™ Training Course for Autonomic Assessment, Interpretation and Clinical Management
- The Nemechek Protocol™ MyHRV Monitoring App
- The Nemechek Protocol™ MyVNS Smart Phone-Enabled Vagus Nerve Stimulator

For more information about certification and licensing:
Info@AutonomicMed.com
Additional Resources:
AutonomicMed.com

AutonomicRecovery.com
@ConcussionFixer

Made in the USA
Monee, IL
21 November 2019